50 MEAL IDEAS FOR AN ALIMENTATION THAT WILL IMPROVE YOUR HEALTH

Amaze Your Friends with These Chef-Life Recipes You Can Re-Create in Your Home Kitchen

Soothing Cooking

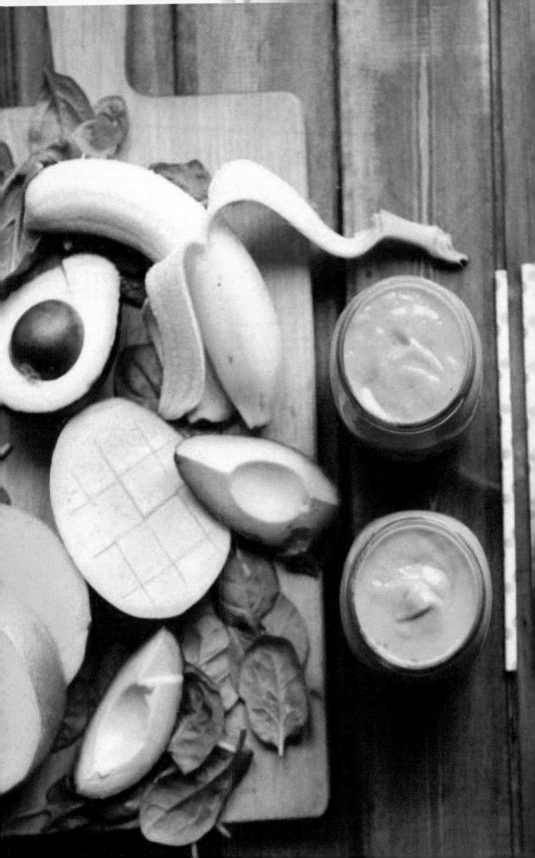

Table of Contents

INTRODUCTION

The Anti-Inflammatory Diet

If you have a condition that causes inflammation, such as chronic peptic, ulcer, asthma, tuberculosis, sinusitis, rheumatoid periodontitis, Crohn's disease, active hepatitis, or arthritis, an anti-inflammatory diet can help. The connection between inflammation and heart disease, arthritis, and other chronic ailments is becoming increasingly clear. Many food allergies and poor dietary choices over stimulate the immune system and cause inflammatory responses that destroy the body's wellness and pave the way for ill health. Inflammation can undermine the overall health of the body, leading to disease down the road and impairing the proper functioning of the brain, joints, cardiovascular system, and skin.

As you will see, the anti-inflammatory diet is simple to follow and is not overly strict. You are able to adjust the diet according to your own preferences. Nevertheless, there are some cons that you should know. The anti-inflammatory diet can be costly as it is recommended that you eat organic food. Likewise, the diet contains a number of allergens, such as nuts, seeds, and soy.

However, eating the right adjusted food will help to eliminate the cons of the diet. It is highly recommended to consult your doctor for a complete medical examination before starting. By doing this, you can avoid unwanted effects of diet.

Ways of Reducing Inflammation Overnight

- Eat salads every day.
- Keep your blood sugar in normal parameters by taking balanced snacks without added sugar and refined carbs.
- Sleep for 7-8 hours every night.
- Take a break from alcohol and add green tea to your routine instead of tea or coffee.
- Go for walk every daily.
- Cut out added sugars and trans fats from your diet and focus on choosing primarily whole and minimally processed foods.

Anti-Inflammatory Foods

- Fruits
- Vegetables
- Legumes
- Beans
- Lentils
- Whole Grains
- Fish
- Olive Oil
- Poultry
- Nuts
- Low-Fat Dairy
- Seeds

It's believed that the antioxidants in brightly colored fruits and vegetables may lessen the effect of free radicals, which damage cells. So try to incorporate more green vegetables and fruits into your diet. To fight inflammation, go for whole, unprocessed foods with no added sugar.

Worst Food for Inflammation

- Processed meat
- Refined sugar
- Alcohol
- Vegetable oils
- Processed fruits
- Saturated fats
- Gluten
- Artificial trans fats
- Artificial preservatives
- White bread
- Cereals
- White pasta
- Juices
- Sodas
- cookies
- Ice cream
- Candies
- Processed and cured meat

You should stay away from ultra-processed foods, like microwaveable dinners, hot dogs, processed meats, dehydrated soups, chicken nuggets, sugary cereals, biscuits, baked goods, and sauces. These foods have little nutritional value and are high in salt, added sugars, and saturated fat. All of these ingredients are associated with promoting inflammation in the body.

Anti-Inflammatory Diet Tips

- You should gradually replace fast food meals with healthful, homemade lunches.
- Replace sodas and other sugary beverages with still or sparkling mineral water
- Take a variety of fruits, vegetables, and healthy snacks.
- Maintain and control your blood sugar levels by avoiding white foods such as sugar, salt, etc.
- Eat food that is rich in probiotics every day. This will improve the gut's microbe barrier. Such foods are fermented vegetables/fruits, miso, sauerkraut, yogurt, kombucha, kimchi, and milk.
- Sleep for 7 to 8 hours.
- For faster treatment, drink antioxidant beverages. Chili pepper thyme, oregano, basil, and curcumin have anti-inflammatory features and serve as natural painkillers.
- Balance your mind by practicing yoga, meditation or biofeedback.
- Make yourself feel healthier by exercising daily.
- Increase the use of green tea instead of coffee and black tea.

Anti-Inflammation Diet Meal Plan for 1 Week

<u>Monday</u>

Breakfast

Steel cut oats with blueberries

Lunch

Mexican chopped salad with creamy avocado dressing

Pineapple ginger smoothie

Dinner

Thai vegetable curry fry

<u>Tuesday</u>

Breakfast

Steel cut oats with blueberries

Lunch

Sautéed mushroom, kale, and egg seasoned with turmeric.

Pineapple ginger smoothie.

Dinner

Salmon cake

Broccoli and green salad

Wednesday

Breakfast

Millet porridge cooked in coconut milk with mango and blueberries.

Lunch

Large salad topped with left over salmon cakes and a balsamic dressing.

Pineapple ginger smoothie

Dinner

Vegetable burger

Baked sweet potatoes

Thursday

Breakfast

Millet porridge cooked in coconut milk with mango and blueberries.

Lunch

Loaded baked sweet potato

Spiced banana almond smoothie

Dinner

Grilled chicken with sautéed spinach

Friday

Breakfast

Cooked quinoa topped with raspberries and toasted walnuts.

Lunch

Large mixed salad with sunny side up egg

Spiced banana almond smoothie

Dinner

Spring barley and quinoa risotto with asparagus and shitake mushrooms

Saturday

Breakfast

Cooked quinoa topped with raspberries and toasted walnuts

Lunch

Lentil vegetable bowl

Dinner

Grilled salmon

Asparagus

Potato

Sunday

Breakfast

Sweet potato pancake with almond butter

Lunch

Lentil vegetable bowl

Dinner

Quinoa stuffed peppers

SOUPS

Delicious Lentil Soup

Servings: 14

Preparation Time: 35 minutes

Per Serving: calories 211, fat 4, fiber 4, carbs 14, protein 6

Ingredients:

- 4 cups chopped yellow onion
- 4 teaspoons ground turmeric
- 3 tablespoons olive oil
- 4 garlic cloves, minced
- 28 ounces coconut milk, unsweetened
- 1 1/2 cups red lentils, rinsed
- 1 teaspoon ground cinnamon
- 6 cups veggie stock
- 3 teaspoons ground cumin
- A pinch of salt and black pepper
- 12 ounces baby spinach
- 4 teaspoons lime juice
- 1/2 teaspoon ground cardamom
- 30 ounces canned tomatoes, chopped

Procedure:

1. First heat up a pot with the olive oil over medium heat, add the garlic and the onion, stir and sauté for 5 minutes.
2. Then add cardamom, cinnamon, cumin and turmeric, stir and cook for 1 minute.
3. Now add tomatoes, coconut milk, lentils, stock, salt and pepper.
4. Stir the soup, bring it to a simmer and cook for 17 minutes.
5. Finally, add the spinach and lime juice, mix and ladle the soup into bowls and serve.

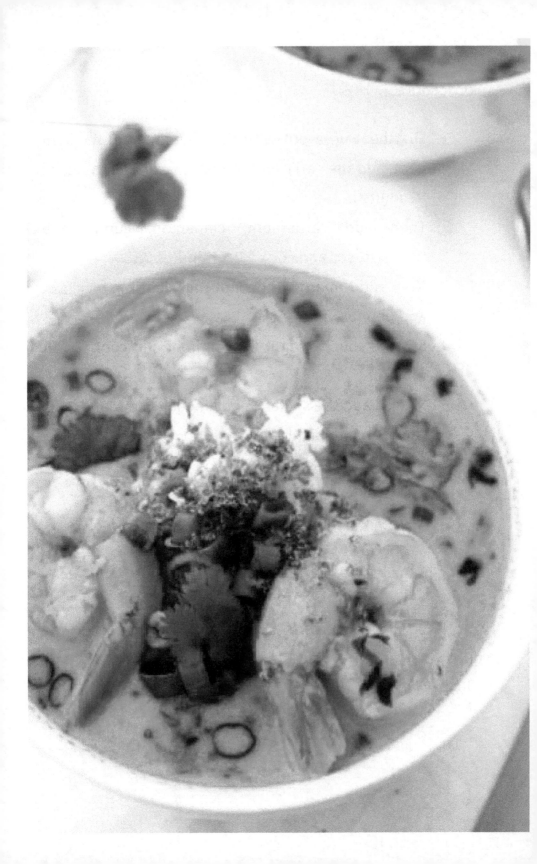

Yummy Shrimp Soup

Servings: 8

Preparation Time: 40 minutes

Per Serving: calories 261, fat 7, fiber 8, carbs 16, protein 11

Ingredients:

- 2 yellow onions, chopped
- 2 pounds mushrooms, sliced
- 4 carrots, sliced
- 12 bok choy heads, torn
- 2 tablespoons olive oil
- 12 garlic cloves, minced
- A pinch of salt and black pepper
- 1 pounds shrimp, deveined and peeled
- 2 teaspoons ground turmeric
- 12 cups chicken stock

Procedure:

1. Firstly, heat up a pot with the oil over medium heat, add the garlic and the onions, stir and sauté for 5 minutes.
2. Then add the stock, carrots, mushrooms, salt, pepper and turmeric.
3. Now bring to a simmer, stir and cook for 20 minutes.
4. In conclusion, add the bok choy and the shrimp, stir and cook for 5 minutes more, then ladle everything into bowls and serve.

Tempting Lemon Lentil Soup

Servings: 6

Preparation Time: 6

Per Serving: calories 271, fat 8, fiber 11, carbs 16, protein 8

Ingredients:

- 1½ cups chopped celery
- 3 garlic cloves, minced
- 1½ cups carrots, sliced
- Juice of 3 small lemons
- 32 ounces veggie stock
- 2 teaspoons ground turmeric
- 1 tablespoon olive oil
- 1 yellow onion, chopped
- 4 teaspoons fresh grated ginger
- 2 cups green lentils, rinsed
- Zest of ½ lemon, grated
- A pinch of salt and black pepper

Procedure:

1. First of all, heat up a pot with the oil over medium heat and add the celery, carrots, onion, a pinch of salt and pepper.
2. Then mix together and sauté for 5 minutes.
3. After that, add the ginger and the garlic, stir and cook for 1 minute more.
4. Now add the lentils, stock and turmeric.
5. Stir, reduce heat to low, cover the pot and cook for 45 minutes.
6. Then add lemon juice and lemon zest, stir and cook the soup for 30 minutes more.
7. Finally, ladle into bowls and serve.

Turkish Style Soup

Servings: 8

Preparation Time: 50 minutes

Per Serving: calories 210, fat 1, fiber 5, carbs 14, protein 6

Ingredients:

- 3 cups cauliflower florets, chopped
- 10 cups vegetable stock
- 4 tablespoons coconut oil, melted
- 8 shallots, chopped
- 8 cups kale, chopped
- Salt and black pepper to the taste
- 2 red bell peppers, chopped
- 30 ounces canned tomatoes, chopped
- 6 carrots, chopped
- 2 pounds ground turkey

Procedure:

1. First, heat up a pot with the oil over medium-high heat.

2. Then add shallots, cauliflower, bell pepper and carrots, stir and cook for 10 minutes.
3. Now add ground turkey, stir and cook for 8 more minutes.
4. Add tomatoes, salt, pepper, kale and stock.
5. Stir, bring to a boil, cover, cook for 15 minutes, then ladle into bowls and serve

Pleasant Ginger Cauliflower Soup

Servings: 8

Preparation Time: 35 minutes

Per Serving: 76 calories, 2.7g protein, 10g carbohydrates, 3.8g fat, 3.9g fiber, 0mg cholesterol, 70mg sodium, 475mg potassium.

Ingredients:

- 2 teaspoons chili powder
- 8 cups of water
- 2 teaspoons ginger, grated
- 1 cup fresh cilantro, chopped
- 2 teaspoons minced garlic
- 2 tablespoons olive oil
- 4 carrots, peeled and grated
- 2 pounds cauliflower, chopped

Procedure:

1. First, pour olive oil into the saucepan.
2. Then add minced garlic, ginger, and chili powder.

3. Stir the mixture and cook it for 2 minutes.

4. Then add all remaining ingredients and carefully stir the soup with the help of the spoon.

5. Finally, cook it for 23 minutes.

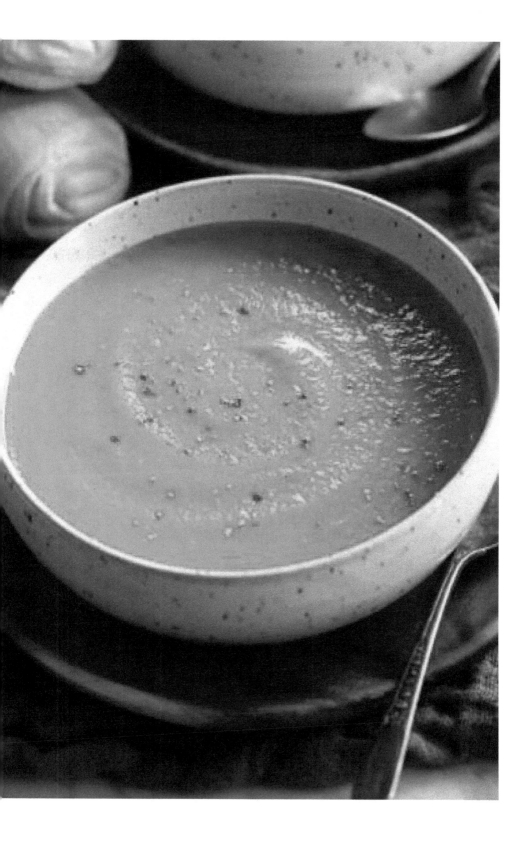

Delicious Tomato Soup

Servings: 8

Preparation Time: 35 minutes

Per Serving: 45 calories, 2.5g protein, 9.4g carbohydrates, 0.6g fat, 3.2g fiber, 0mg cholesterol, 23mg sodium, 545mg potassium.

Ingredients:

- 2 teaspoons cayenne pepper
- 8 cups tomatoes, chopped
- 2 teaspoons garlic, diced
- 2 cups broccoli, chopped
- 4 cups of water
- 2 teaspoons ground paprika
- 1 cup fresh spinach, chopped

Directions:

1. First of all, put all ingredients in the saucepan and close the lid.

2. Then simmer the soup for 20 minutes on the medium heat.

3. Now blend the soup with the help of the immersion blender.

4. Finally, bring the cream soup to boil and cook for 5 minutes more.

Heavenly Green Soup

Servings: 8

Preparation Time: 30 minutes

Per Serving: 90 calories, 4.7g protein, 11.5g carbohydrates, 4.2g fat, 4.6g fiber, 0mg cholesterol, 105mg sodium, 977mg potassium.

Ingredients:

- 8 cups of water
- 8 cherry tomatoes, halved
- 2 pounds spinach, chopped
- 2 yellow onions, chopped
- 1 cup fresh cilantro, chopped
- 2 tablespoons olive oil

Procedure:

1. Firstly, pour the olive oil into the saucepan.
2. Secondly, add onions and roast them for 2-3 minutes.
3. Then add spinach, tomatoes, and fresh cilantro.
4. Now close the lid and cook the soup on medium heat for 18 minutes.

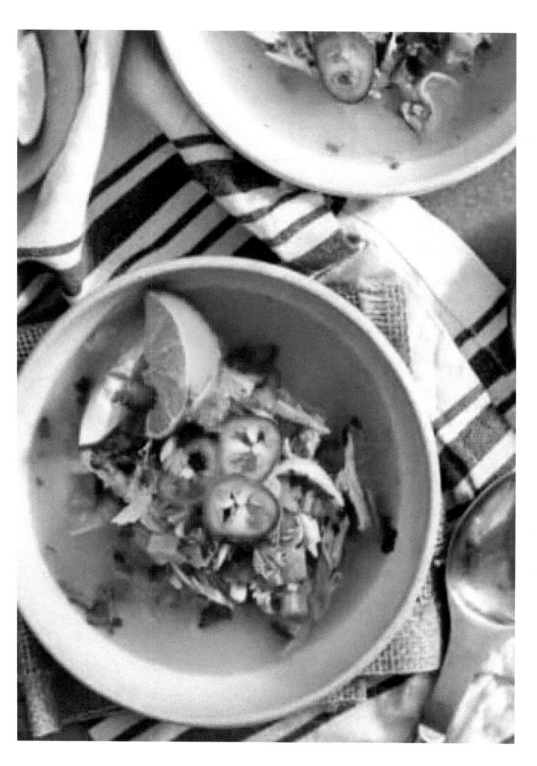

Delectable Chicken Soup With lime

Servings: 8

Preparation Time: 1 hour

Per Serving: calories 271, fat 8, fiber 11, carbs 16, protein 8

Ingredients:

- 3 garlic cloves, minced
- A pinch of salt and black pepper
- 1 yellow onion, chopped
- 1 pound chicken breast, skinless, boneless and cubed
- 1 tablespoon olive oil
- Juice of 1 lime
- Zest of 1 lime, grated
- 1 tablespoon cilantro, chopped
- 2 carrots, sliced
- 6 cups veggie stock
- 2 teaspoons turmeric powder

Procedure:

1. First, heat up a pot with the oil over medium heat, add the onion, carrots and garlic and sauté for 5 minutes.
2. Then add the meat and brown it for 5 minutes more.
3. Now add the stock and the other ingredients except the cilantro, toss, bring to a simmer and cook over medium heat for 50 minutes.
4. Divide the soup into bowls, sprinkle the cilantro on top and serve.

Pleasant Veggie Carrot Soup

Servings: 4

Preparation Time: 35 minutes

Per Serving: calories 210, fat 8, fiber 6, carbs 10, protein 7

Ingredients:

- 1 teaspoon rosemary, dried
- 1 teaspoon cumin, ground
- ½ teaspoon turmeric powder
- 1 pound carrots, peeled and sliced
- 2 tablespoons olive oil
- 1 yellow onion, chopped
- 2 garlic cloves, minced
- 1 cup coconut milk
- 1 tablespoon chives, chopped
- A pinch of salt and black pepper
- 5 cups vegetable stock

Procedure:

1. First, heat up a pot with the oil over medium heat, add the onion and the garlic and sauté for 5 minutes.
2. Then add the carrots, the stock and the other ingredients except the chives, stir, bring to a simmer and cook over medium heat for 20 minutes more.
3. Now divide the soup into bowls, sprinkle the chives on top and serve for lunch.

Flavorful Vegetable Artichoke Soup

Servings: 8

Preparation Time: 35 minutes

Per Serving: calories 200, fat 4, fiber 4, carbs 12, protein 8

Ingredients:

- 4 tomatoes, cubed
- 4 tablespoons olive oil
- 2 teaspoons cumin, ground
- 2 tablespoons rosemary, chopped
- 4 yellow onions, chopped
- 1/2 teaspoon turmeric powder
- 4 cups canned artichoke hearts, drained and halved
- A pinch of salt and black pepper
- 10 cups vegetable stock
- 2 tablespoons tomato paste

Procedure:

1. First, heat up a pot with the oil over medium-high heat, add the onions and sauté for 5 minutes.

34

2. Then add the artichokes and the other ingredients toss bring to a simmer and cook over medium heat for 25 minutes more.

3. Now ladle the soup into bowls and serve.

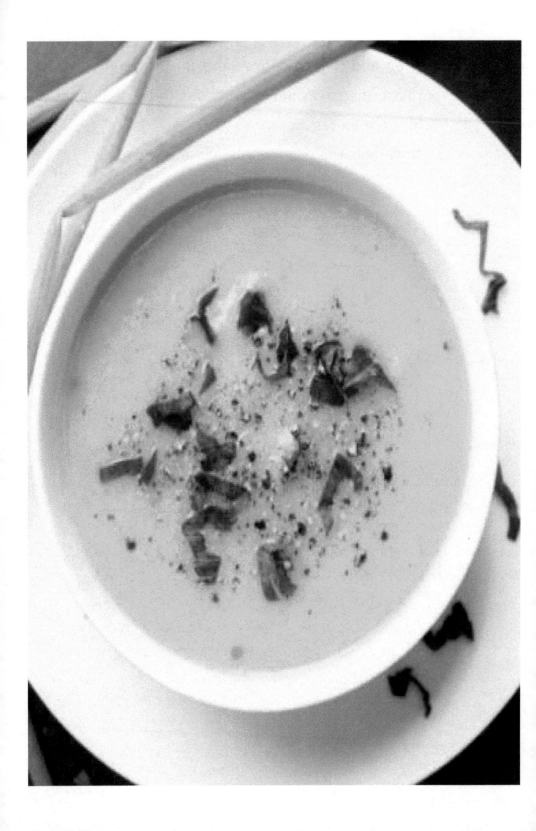

Tempting Veggie Leeks Soup

Servings: 8

Preparation Time: 30 minutes

Per Serving: calories 268, fat 11.8, fiber 4.5, carbs 37.4, protein 6.1

Ingredients:

- 8 leeks, sliced
- 2 yellow onions, chopped
- 1 teaspoon nutmeg, ground
- 1/2 teaspoon red pepper, crushed
- 4 garlic cloves, minced
- 8 cups vegetable soup
- 1 cup coconut milk
- 2 tablespoons avocado oil
- A pinch of salt and black pepper
- 2 tablespoons parsley, chopped
- 1 teaspoon rosemary, dried

Procedure:

1. First, heat up a pot with the oil over medium-high heat, add the onion and the garlic and sauté for 2 minutes.
2. Then add the leeks, stir and sauté for 3 minutes more.
3. Now add the stock and the rest of the ingredients except the parsley, bring to a simmer and cook over medium heat for 15 minutes more.
4. Finally, blend the soup with an immersion blender, divide the soup into bowls, sprinkle the parsley on top and serve.

Delightful Chicken Soup

Servings: 12

Preparation Time: 25 minutes

Per Serving: calories 210, fat 7, fiber 2, carbs 10, protein 8

Ingredients:

- 2 bunches kale, chopped
- 6 carrots, chopped
- 2 tablespoons chopped parsley
- Salt and black pepper to the taste
- 2 cups cooked shredded chicken
- 2 cups white mushrooms, sliced
- 4 quarts vegetable stock

Procedure:

1. Initially, heat up a pot with the stock over medium heat, add carrots, mushrooms, chicken, kale, salt and pepper.
2. Then stir the soup, bring to a simmer and cook for 15 minutes. Ladle into bowls and serve for lunch.

39

Enjoyable Chicken Soup

Servings: 8

Preparation Time: 1 hour

Per Serving: calories 211, fat 4, fiber 7, carbs 13, protein 8

Ingredients:

- 5 garlic cloves, minced
- 8 cups chicken stock
- 2 tablespoons olive oil
- 2 celery stalks, chopped
- 3 tablespoons chopped parsley
- 2 tablespoons lemon juice
- 2 tablespoons chopped dill
- 2 carrots, chopped
- 2½ pounds chicken thighs, boneless and skinless
- 1 yellow onion, chopped
- A pinch of salt and black pepper

Procedure:

1. First, heat up a soup pot with the oil over medium-high heat.
2. Add the celery, onion, carrots, and garlic, then stir and cook for 10 minutes.
3. Now add the chicken, stock, salt and pepper, stir, then bring to a boil and reduce heat to medium-low.
4. Then cover and cook for 40 minutes.
5. Transfer the chicken to a cutting board, shred the meat, discard bones and return the shredded chicken to the pot.
6. Finally, cook everything for 4-5 minutes more, add parsley, dill and lemon juice, then toss, ladle into bowls and serve.

SNACKS & SIDE DISHES

Coconut Zucchini Lunch Cream

Servings: 8

Preparation Time: 35 minutes

Per Serving: calories 312, fat 9, fiber 2, carbs 34, protein 7

Ingredients:

- 4 tablespoons coconut milk
- 4 garlic cloves, minced
- 2 onions, chopped
- 6 zucchinis, cut into medium chunks
- A pinch of sea salt and black pepper
- 8 cups chicken stock
- 4 tablespoons olive oil

Procedure:

1. First, heat up a pot with the oil over medium heat.
2. Then add zucchinis, garlic and onion, stir and cook for 5 minutes.
3. Add stock, salt and pepper, then stir.

4. Now bring to a boil, cover the pot and simmer the soup for 20 minutes.

5. Mix with the coconut milk, blend using an immersion blender, ladle into bowls and serve.

Chicken & Pumpkin Stew

Servings: 6

Preparation Time: 8 hours 10 minutes

Per Serving: calories 280, fat 3, fiber 3, carbs 6, protein 7

Ingredients:

- 2 quarts chicken stock
- 2 cups chicken meat, skinless, boneless and shredded
- 2 carrots, chopped
- 5 garlic cloves, minced
- 2 celery sticks, chopped
- ¼ teaspoon cayenne pepper
- ¼ cup ground arrowroot
- 2 onions, chopped
- 2 sweet potatoes, cubed
- 30 ounces canned pumpkin puree
- ½ pound baby spinach
- A pinch of sea salt and black pepper

Procedure:

1. Take your slow cooker, mix carrots with garlic, celery, onion, sweet potatoes, pumpkin puree, chicken, stock, salt, pepper, cayenne and ground arrowroot.
2. Stir, cover and cook on Low for 8 hours.
3. Then uncover slow cooker, add spinach, stir, divide the stew into bowls and serve.

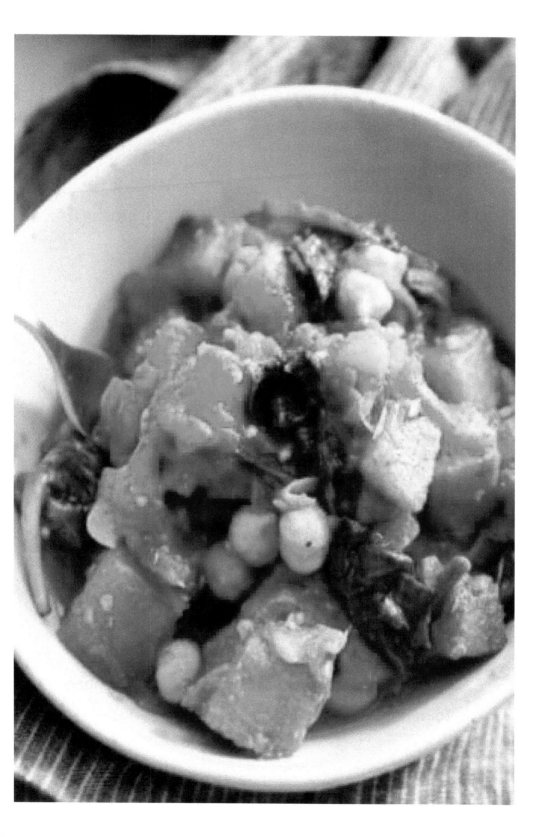

Eggplant & Tomato Lunch Stew

Servings: 35 minutes

Preparation Time: 6

Per Serving: calories 210, fat 5, fiber 5, carbs 14, protein 8

Ingredients:

- A pinch of cayenne pepper
- 2 teaspoons ground cumin
- 4 big tomatoes, chopped
- 2 eggplants, chopped
- 2 cups tomatoes paste
- 1 cup vegetable stock
- 2 yellow onions, chopped
- A pinch of salt and black pepper

Procedure:

1. First, put the stock in a small pot and heat it up over medium heat.
2. Then add the tomato paste, cayenne, salt, pepper, tomatoes, eggplant and onion.

3. Stir, bring to a simmer, cover the pot and cook the stew for 25 minutes.
4. Divide into bowls and serve.

Flavorful Lemony Salmon

Servings: 4

Preparation Time: 1 hour 10 minutes

Per Serving: calories 200, fat 8, fiber 3, carbs 6, protein 10

Ingredients:

- 4 teaspoons olive oil
- A pinch of salt and black pepper
- 2 big salmon fillets, halved

For the relish:

- 2 Meyer lemons, cut in wedges and then thinly sliced
- 4 tablespoons parsley, chopped
- 2 tablespoons lemon juice
- 2 shallots, chopped
- 1/2 cup olive oil

Procedure:

1. Arrange the salmon on a lined baking dish, drizzle 4 teaspoons olive oil, season with sea salt and black pepper and rub the seasoning into the fish.
2. Place in the oven at 370 degrees F and bake for 1 hour.
3. In a bowl, mix shallot with the lemon juice, salt and black pepper, stir and leave aside for 10 minutes.
4. In another bowl, whisk together the marinated shallot with lemon slices, some salt, pepper, parsley and ¼ cup oil.
5. Cut salmon in chunks, divide between plates, top with lemon relish and serve.

Cod Fillets

Servings: 4

Preparation Time: 30 minutes

Per Serving: calories 210, fat 12, fiber 6, carbs 9, protein 12

Ingredients:

- 2 garlic cloves, minced
- 2 tablespoons lemon juice
- 1 tablespoon chopped parsley
- 4 medium cod filets
- 1 teaspoon Dijon mustard
- 1 shallot, chopped
- A pinch of salt and black pepper
- ¼ cup oil+ 2 tablespoons

Procedure:

1. Take a bowl, whisk together the mustard with ¼ cup oil, garlic, parsley, shallot, lemon juice, salt and pepper. Heat up a pan with the rest of the oil over medium-high heat.

2. Add fish fillets, season them with salt and black pepper and cook for 4 minutes on each side.
3. Spread mustard mix over the fish, transfer everything to a lined baking sheet and place in the oven at 425 degrees F.
4. Bake for 10 minutes, divide between plates and serve with a side salad

Tempting Lemon Turkey

Servings: 8

Preparation Time: 40 minutes

Per Serving: 154 calories, 24g protein, 4.1g carbohydrates, 4.9g fat, 0.5g fiber, 0mg cholesterol, 0mg sodium, 29mg potassium

Ingredients:

- 2 teaspoons cayenne pepper
- 2-pounds turkey fillet, chopped
- 2 tablespoons olive oil
- 2 lemons

Procedure:

1. First of all, mix the turkey fillet with cayenne pepper and olive oil.
2. Then squeeze the lemon in the turkey and transfer the meal into the baking tray.
3. Bake the turkey at 360F for 30 minutes.

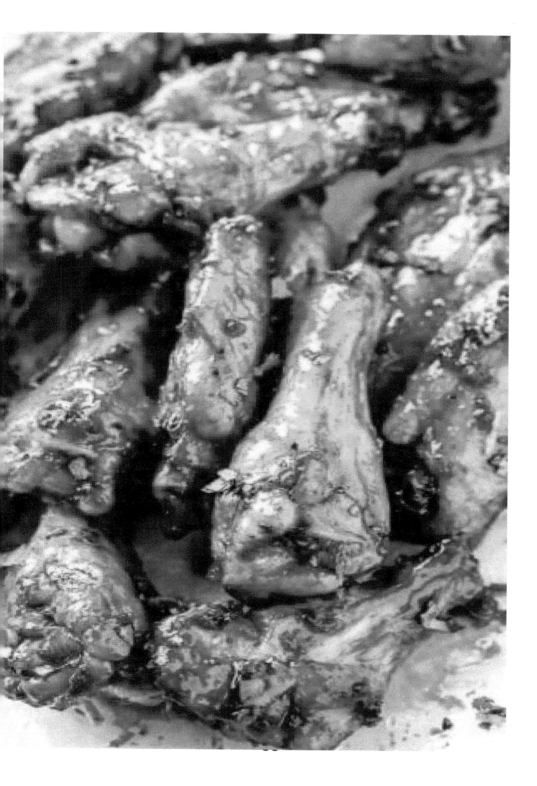

Delicious Honey Chicken Wings

Servings: 8

Preparation Time: 1 hour 10 minutes

Per Serving: 466 calories, 65.8g protein, 9.1g carbohydrates, 17g fat, 0.3g fiber, 202mg cholesterol, 203mg sodium, 574mg potassium

Ingredients:

- 2 teaspoons chili powder
- 2 tablespoons lemon juice
- 4 pounds chicken wings, halved
- 4 tablespoons raw honey

Procedure:

1. First, mix chicken wings with raw honey, chili powder, and lemon juice.
2. Then wrap the chicken wings in the foil and put it in the tray.
3. Bake the chicken wings at 350F for 1 hour.

Wrapped Chicken

Servings: 8

Preparation Time: 30 minutes

Per Serving: 193 calories, 22g protein, 6.5g carbohydrates, 8.8g fat, 1.2g fiber, 62mg cholesterol, 86mg sodium, 462mg potassium

Ingredients:

- 16 oz kale leaves
- 1 cup of water
- 4 cups ground chicken
- 2 teaspoons ground black pepper
- 2 teaspoons dried oregano
- 2 tablespoons olive oil

Procedure:

1. First, pour olive oil into the skillet.
2. Add dried oregano, ground black pepper, and ground chicken.
3. Cook the mixture for 10 minutes.

4. Then put the chicken mixture on the kale leaves and wrap them.
5. Put the wrapped kale in the skillet, add water.
6. Close the lid and cook the meal on medium heat for 10 minutes.

Squash & Garlic Shrimp

Servings: 8

Preparation Time: 20 minutes

Per Serving: calories 211, fat 6, fiber 4, carbs 11, protein 8

Ingredients:

- 2 pounds shrimp, peeled and deveined
- 4 tablespoons pine nuts
- 2 yellow squashes, peeled and cubed
- 4 tablespoons olive oil
- 8 scallions, chopped
- 4 garlic cloves, minced
- 4 tablespoons chives, chopped

Procedure:

1. First, heat up a pan with the oil over medium heat, add the scallions and the garlic and sauté for 2 minutes.

2. Then add the shrimp and the other ingredients, toss, cook everything for 10 minutes more, divide into bowls and serve for lunch.

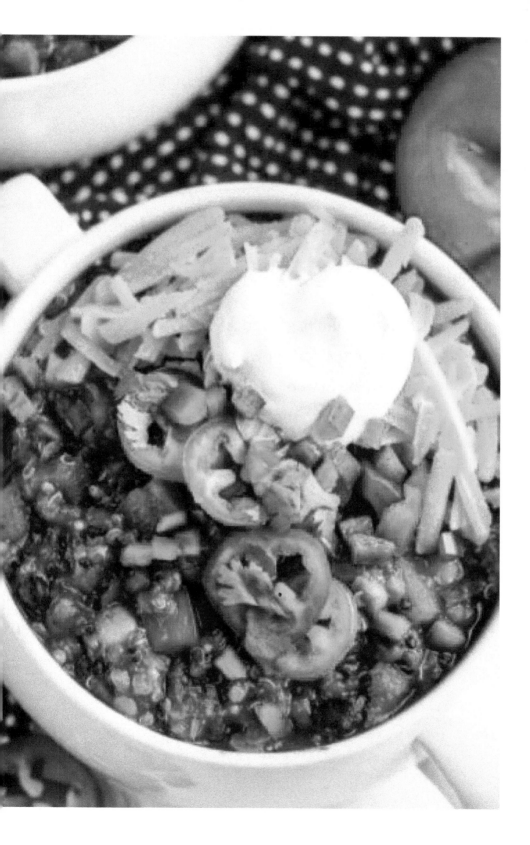

Zucchini & Chili Quinoa Mix

Servings: 4

Preparation Time: 30 minutes

Per Serving: calories 182, fat 2, fiber 4, carbs 8, protein 11

Ingredients:

- 1 teaspoon cumin, ground
- 1 teaspoon turmeric powder
- 1 tablespoon olive oil
- 1 yellow onion, chopped
- 2 garlic cloves, minced
- 3 tablespoons coconut aminos
- 1 teaspoon chili powder
- 1 cup quinoa, cooked
- 2 zucchinis, sliced
- 1 tablespoon ginger, grated
- 1 tablespoon hemp seeds

Procedure:

1. First, heat up a pan with the oil over medium heat, add the onion and the garlic and sauté for 5 minutes.
2. Then add the quinoa, the zucchinis and the other ingredients, toss, cook everything for 15 minutes more, divide into bowls and serve for lunch.

Healthy Chicken Soup with Chard

Servings: 8

Preparation Time: 40 minutes

Per Serving: calories 181, fat 4, fiber 4, carbs 9, protein 11

Ingredients:

- 1 teaspoon red chili flakes
- A pinch of salt and black pepper
- 2 yellow onions, chopped
- 4 tablespoons olive oil
- 4 garlic cloves, minced
- 2 pounds chicken thighs, skinless, boneless and cubed
- 1 teaspoon turmeric powder
- 12 cups veggie stock
- 2 bunches chard, roughly chopped
- 2 tablespoons cilantro, chopped

Procedure:

1. First, heat up a pot with the oil over medium heat, add the onion and the garlic and sauté for 5 minutes.
2. Then add the meat and brown for 5 minutes more.
3. Add the stock and the other ingredients, toss, bring to a simmer and cook over medium heat for 20 minutes more.
4. Finally, divide the soup into bowls and serve.

Lemon Salmon with Peaches

Servings: 8

Preparation Time: 25 minutes

Per Serving: calories 211, fat 4, fiber 8, carbs 16, protein 7

Ingredients:

- 2 cups peaches, cubed
- 2 tablespoons lemon juice
- 2 bunches kale, torn
- 8 scallions, chopped
- 4 garlic cloves, minced
- 2 tablespoons olive oil
- 2 pounds salmon fillets, boneless and cut into strips
- 2 tablespoons pine nuts.
- A pinch of salt and black pepper
- 1 tablespoon balsamic vinegar

Procedure:

1. First, heat up a pan with the oil over medium heat, add the scallions and the garlic and sauté for 2 minutes.
2. Then add the salmon and cook for 5 minutes more.
3. Add the rest of the ingredients, toss gently, cook everything for 13 minutes more, divide into bowls and serve for lunch.

Chard & Sesame Spread

Servings: 8

Preparation Time: 20 minutes

Per Serving: calories 142, fat 6, fiber 3, carbs 7, protein 4

Ingredients:

- 4 teaspoons olive oil
- 4 garlic cloves, minced
- 4 cups Swiss chard leaves
- Juice of 2 limes
- 2 tablespoons chopped cilantro
- 1 cup veggie stock
- ½ cup sesame paste
- A pinch of salt and black pepper

Procedure:

1. First, put the stock in a small pot and bring it to a simmer over medium heat.
2. Then add the Swiss chard, salt and pepper to the pot, bring to a simmer and cook for about 10 minutes.

3. Now drain and put in a food processor along with the garlic, sesame paste, lime juice, olive oil and cilantro.
4. Pulse well, divide into bowls and serve.

<u>LUNCH</u>

Peanut Butter Dip

Servings: 8

Preparation Time: 10 minutes

Per Serving: calories 110, fat 1, fiber 5, carbs 7, protein 5

Ingredients:

- 1 cup coconut cream
- 1 cup peanut butter, soft

Procedure:

1. Take a bowl, whisk together the peanut butter with the coconut cream. Divide into bowls and serve.

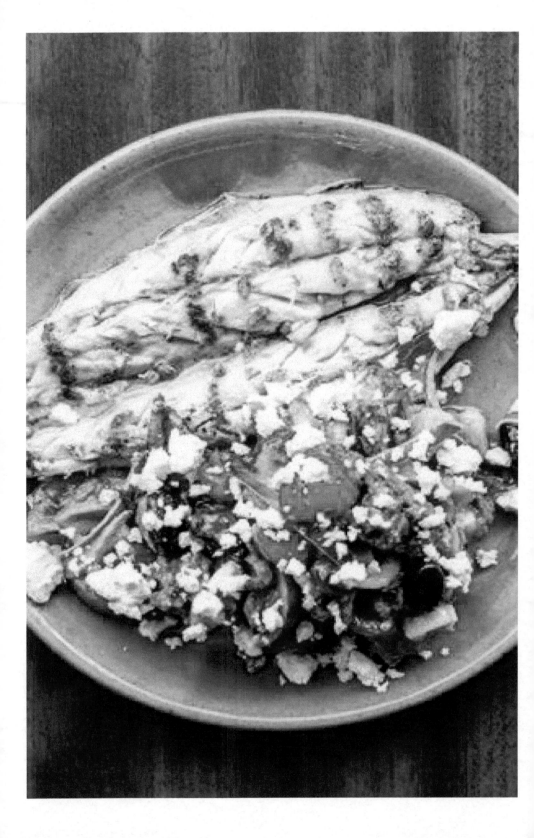

Oregano Sea Bass with Tomatoes

Servings: 4

Preparation Time: 25 minutes

Per Serving: calories 273, fat 6, fiber 6, carbs 10, protein 11

Ingredients:

- 1 tablespoon lemon juice
- 1 tablespoon oregano, chopped
- 4 sea bass fillets, boneless
- 1 yellow onion, chopped
- 2 tablespoons olive oil
- 1 cup cherry tomatoes, halved
- 1 tablespoon chives, chopped
- 2 garlic cloves, chopped
- Salt and black pepper to the taste

Procedure:

1. First, heat up a pan with the oil over medium heat, add the onion and the garlic and sauté for 2 minutes.

2. Then add the fish and sear it for 2 minutes on each
   side.
3. Add the rest of the ingredients, cook everything for
   14 minutes more, divide between plates and serve.

Nutmeg Apple Snack

Servings: 8

Preparation Time: 2 hours 10 minutes

Per Serving: calories 141, fat 2, fiber 2, carbs 7, protein 5

Ingredients:

- Ground Cinnamon to taste
- 4 apples, cored and cubed
- Cooking spray
- A pinch of ground nutmeg

Procedure:

1. First, arrange the apple cubes on a lined baking sheet and sprinkle with cinnamon, nutmeg and spray with the cooking oil.
2. Then toss the apple slices well and place in the oven at 275 degrees F.
3. Bake for 2 hours.
4. Divide into bowls and serve as a snack

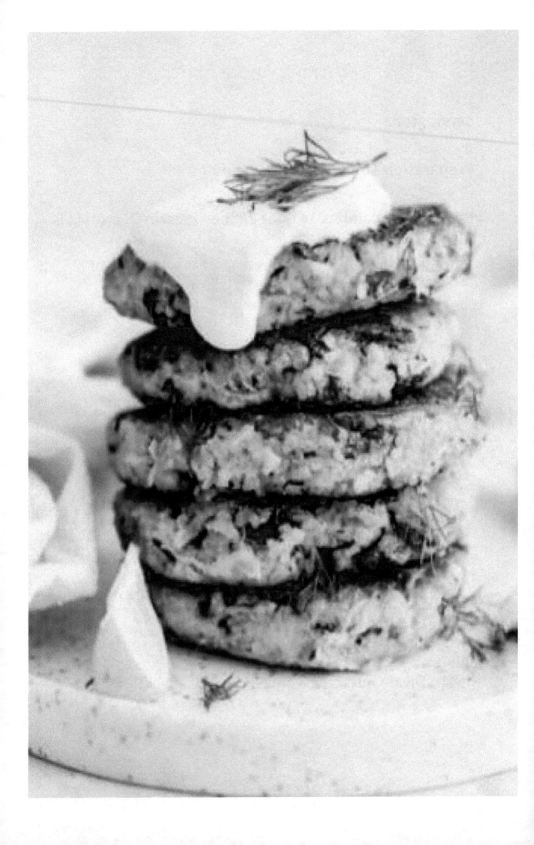

Delicious Dill Zucchini Patties

Servings: 12

Preparation Time: 30 minutes

Per Serving: calories 120, fat 4, fiber 2, carbs 6, protein 6

Ingredients:

- ½ cup coconut flour
- A pinch of sea salt and black pepper
- Cooking spray
- 2 garlic cloves, minced
- 3 zucchinis, grated and excess water squeezed
- ½ cup chopped dill
- 1 egg
- 1 yellow onion, chopped

Procedure:

1. Take a bowl, mix zucchinis with garlic, onion, flour, salt, pepper, egg and dill.
2. Then shape medium patties out of this mix and arrange them on a lined baking sheet.

3. Now spray them with cooking oil, and bake in the oven at 400 degrees F for 10 minutes on each side.

4. Arrange the patties on a platter and serve as an appetizer.

Spiralized Carrot

Servings: 8

Preparation Time: 10 minutes

Per Serving: 77 calories, 1g protein, 11.4g carbohydrates, 3.5g fat, 2.8g fiber, 0mg cholesterol, 75mg sodium, 354mg potassium.

Ingredients:

- 2 tablespoons olive oil
- 2 teaspoons ground black pepper
- 14 carrots, spiralized
- 4 tablespoons lime juice

Procedure:

1. First, preheat the olive oil in the skillet well.
2. Add carrot and ground black pepper.
3. Then roast the carrot for 2-3 minutes.
4. Add lime juice, stir the carrot, and cook it for 2 minutes more.

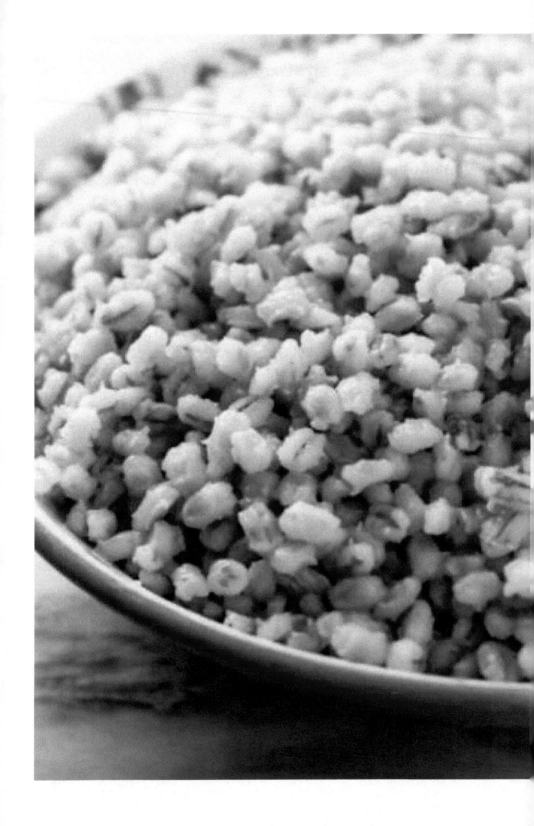

Classic Barley

Servings: 8

Preparation Time: 35 minutes

Per Serving: 356 calories, 11.5g protein, 67.6g carbohydrates, 5.6g fat, 15.9g fiber, 0mg cholesterol, 18mg sodium, 418mg potassium.

Ingredients:

- 2 tablespoons olive oil
- 4 cups barley
- 8 cups of water

Procedure:

1. Mix water with barley and olive oil.
2. Cook the barley with the closed lid for 30 minutes on low heat.

Cabbage Slaw

Servings: 8

Preparation Time: 10 minutes

Per Serving: 83 calories, 1g protein, 9.4g carbohydrates, 5.4g fat, 1.7g fiber, 0mg cholesterol, 19mg sodium, 184mg potassium.

Ingredients:

- 6 tablespoons raisins, chopped
- 4 tablespoons coconut cream
- 4 cups green cabbage, shredded
- 2 tablespoons lemon juice
- 2 tablespoons olive oil
- 2 carrots, grated

Procedure:

1. First, mix green cabbage with carrot, raisins, coconut cream, and lemon juice.
2. Then add olive oil and carefully mix the slaw.

Mushroom Coconut Spread

Servings: 8

Preparation Time: 35 minutes

Per Serving: calories 120, fat 8, fiber 5, carbs 10, protein 9

Ingredients:

- 1 teaspoon turmeric powder
- 1 teaspoon coriander, ground
- 1 tablespoon olive oil
- 1 yellow onion, chopped
- A pinch of salt and black pepper
- 1 tablespoon dill, chopped
- 1 pound white mushrooms, sliced
- 3 garlic cloves, minced
- 2 cups coconut cream

Procedure:

1. Heat up a pan with the oil over medium heat, add the onion and the garlic and sauté for 5 minutes.
2. Add the mushrooms and sauté for 5 minutes more.

3. Add the rest of the ingredients, stir, cook over medium heat for 15 minutes, blend using an immersion blender, divide into bowls and serve.

Spinach Dip Sauce

Servings: 12

Preparation Time: 10 minutes

Per Serving: calories 120, fat 12, fiber 2, carbs 11, protein 5

Ingredients:

- Juice of 2 limes
- 1 teaspoon cumin, ground
- 2 cups coconut cream
- A pinch of salt and black pepper
- 6 garlic cloves, chopped
- 4 tablespoons cilantro, chopped
- 1 cup baby spinach

Procedure:

1. Take your blender, combine the cream with the cilantro and the other ingredients, pulse, divide into bowls and serve as a party dip.

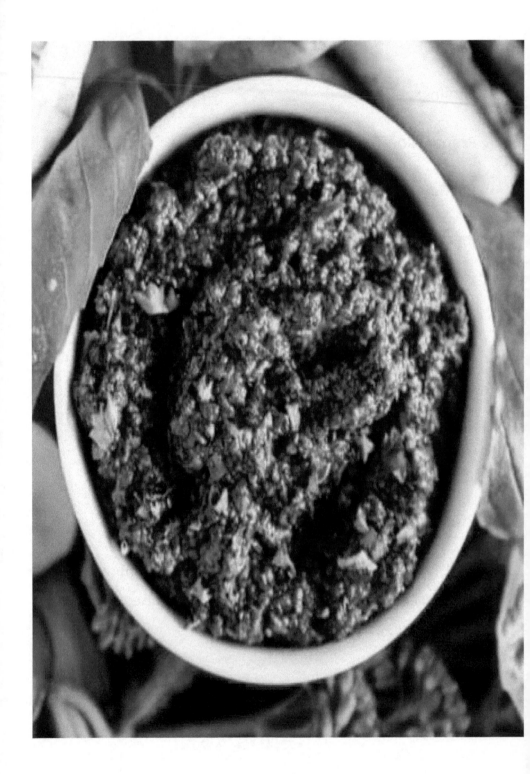

Olives Tapenade

Servings: 8

Preparation Time: 10 minutes

Per Serving: calories 165, fat 11, fiber 4, carbs 8, protein 5

Ingredients:

- 4 tablespoons olive oil
- 4 garlic cloves, chopped
- 2 cups black olives, pitted and sliced
- A pinch of salt and black pepper
- Juice of 1 lime
- 1 tablespoon cilantro, chopped

Procedure:

1. Take a blender, combine the olives with salt, pepper and the other ingredients, pulse well, divide into small bowls and serve as a party dip.

Cilantro Bok Choy Dip

Servings: 12

Preparation Time: 35 minutes

Per Serving: calories 150, fat 2, fiber 3, carbs 8, protein 5

Ingredients:

- 2 cups coconut cream
- 2 tablespoons olive oil
- 4 garlic cloves, minced
- 2 tablespoons cilantro, chopped
- A pinch of salt and black pepper
- 2 pounds bok choy, torn
- 2 yellow onions, chopped

Procedure:

1. First, heat up a pan with the oil over medium heat, add the onion and the garlic and sauté for 5 minutes.
2. Then add the rest of the ingredients, stir, cook over medium heat for 20 minutes, blend using an immersion blender, divide into bowls and serve.

Walnut Baked Snack

Servings: 8

Preparation Time: 24 minutes

Per Serving: calories 100, fat 2, fiber 4, carbs 11, protein 6

Ingredients:

- 2 teaspoons smoked paprika
- 2 cups walnuts
- A pinch of salt and black pepper
- 2 tablespoons olive oil
- 2 teaspoons garlic powder

Procedure:

1. First, spread the walnuts on a baking sheet lined with parchment paper, add the oil and the other ingredients, toss and bake at 400 degrees F for 14 minutes.
2. Then divide the mix into bowls and serve.

SMOOTHIES

Blackberries & Spinach Smoothie

Servings: 2

Preparation Time: 10 minutes

Per Serving: calories 160, fat 3, fiber 4, carbs 6, protein 3

Ingredients:

- 1 banana, peeled and roughly chopped
- 1 cup baby spinach
- 1 cup blackberries
- 1 avocado, pitted, peeled and chopped
- 1 cup water
- ½ cup almond milk, unsweetened
- 1 tablespoon hemp seeds

Procedure:

1. Take your blender; mix the berries with the avocado, banana, spinach, hemp seeds, water and almond milk.
2. Pulse well, divide into 2 glasses and serve for breakfast.

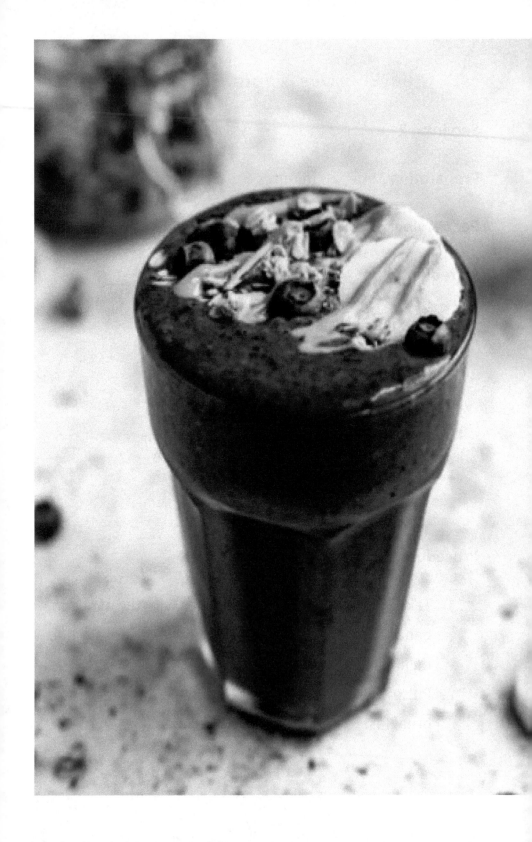

Blackberry Peanut Smoothie

Servings: 2

Preparation Time: 5 minutes

Per Serving: calories 120, fat 3, fiber 3, carbs 6, protein 8

Ingredients:

- 2 tablespoons peanut butter
- 1 1/2 cups almond milk
- 1 1/2 cups blackberries
- 1 banana, peeled
- 4 dates, pitted

Procedure:

1. Take your blender, puree the blackberries with peanut butter, almond milk, banana and dates.
2. Transfer to a bowl and serve cold.

Beet & Mint Smoothie

Servings: 4

Preparation Time: 10 minutes

Per Serving: 76 calories, 3g protein, 17.2g carbohydrates, 0.3g fat, 3.6g fiber, 0mg cholesterol, 135mg sodium, 533mg potassium.

Ingredients:

- 2 tablespoons fresh mint
- 4 cups beets, chopped
- 2 cups of water

Procedure:

1. Put all ingredients in the blender and blend until smooth.

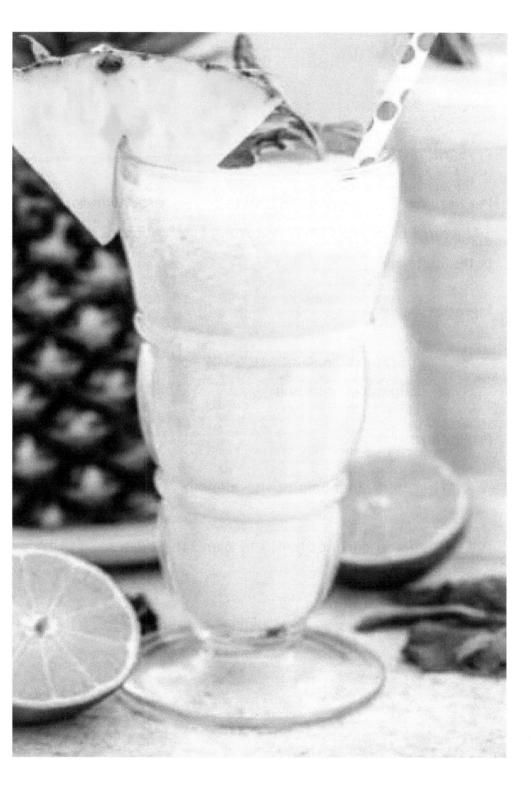

Pineapple Smoothie

Servings: 2

Preparation Time: 10 minutes

Per Serving: 220 calories, 2.3g protein, 25g carbohydrates, 14.5g fat, 3.6g fiber, 0mg cholesterol, 11mg sodium, 338mg potassium.

Ingredients:

- 2 cups pineapple, chopped
- 1/2 cup of coconut milk

Procedure:

1. First, put pineapple in the blender and blend until smooth.
2. Then add coconut milk and blend the mixture until homogenous.

Zucchini Simple Smoothie

Servings: 4

Preparation Time: 10 minutes

Per Serving: 21 calories, 1.5g protein, 4.4g carbohydrates, 0.3g fat, 1.6g fiber, 0mg cholesterol, 15mg sodium, 322mg potassium.

Ingredients:

- 2 cups of water
- 4 cups zucchini, chopped
- 2 teaspoons ground paprika

Procedure:

1. First, blend the zucchini until smooth.
2. Then add water and ground paprika.
3. Now pulse the smoothies for 10 seconds.

Raspberry Smoothie

Servings: 4

Preparation Time: 10 minutes

Per Serving: 102 calories,2.1g protein, 25.3g carbohydrates, 0.4g fat, 6.4g fiber, 0mg cholesterol, 2mg sodium, 380mg potassium.

Ingredients:

- 1 cup of water
- 4 oranges, peeled, chopped
- 1 cup raspberries

Procedure:

1. Blend the raspberries with oranges until smooth.
2. Then add water and blend the mixture for 5 seconds more.

Banana & Raspberry Smoothie

Servings: 2

Preparation Time: 5 minutes

Per Serving: calories 431, fat 34.6, fiber 13.9, carbs 33.3, protein 5.1

Ingredients:

- ½ cup almond milk
- ¼ cup water
- 1 cup baby spinach
- 1 avocado, peeled, pitted and mashed
- 1 banana, peeled and sliced
- 1 cup raspberries

Procedure:

1. Take a blender, combine the spinach with the avocado, and the other ingredients, pulse well, divide into 2 glasses and serve for breakfast.

Banana & Cherries Smoothie

Servings: 4

Preparation Time: 5 minutes

Per Serving: calories 678, fat 81.3, fiber 6.6, carbs 35.5, protein 7.3

Ingredients:

- 1 banana, peeled and frozen
- 4 cups almond milk
- 2 cups cherries, pitted
- 2 tablespoons coconut butter

Procedure:

1. Take your blender, combine the milk with the cherries and the other ingredients, pulse well, divide into glasses and serve.

Banana & Avocado Smoothie

Servings: 2

Preparation Time: 5 minutes

Per Serving: calories 125, fat 6, fiber 7, carbs 9, protein 4

Ingredients:

- 1 cup water
- 1 banana, peeled and mashed
- 1 avocado, pitted and peeled
- 1 cup coconut milk
- 1 cup baby spinach
- 1 tablespoon lime juice

Procedure:

1. Take your blender, combine the avocados with the milk, the water and the remaining ingredients, pulse well, divide into bowls and serve.

Simple Orange Mango Smoothie

Servings: 4

Preparation Time: 10 minutes

Per Serving: calories 100, fat 1, fiber 2, carbs 4, protein 5

Ingredients:

- 2 cups orange juice
- 2 tablespoons ginger, grated
- 4 cups mango, peeled and chopped
- 2 teaspoons turmeric powder

Procedure:

1. Take your blender, combine the mango with the juice and the other ingredients, pulse well, divide into glasses and serve cold.

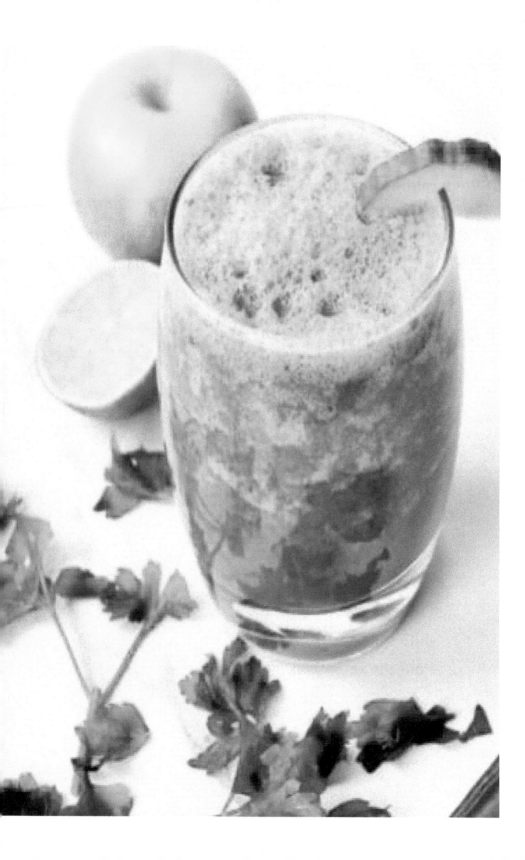

Fresh Parsley Smoothie

Servings: 10

Preparation Time: 10 minutes

Per Serving: 36 calories,1.8g protein, 7.6g carbohydrates, 0.5g fat, 2.5g fiber, 0mg cholesterol, 30mg sodium, 311mg potassium.

Ingredients:

- 2 cups of water
- 2 teaspoons ground black pepper
- 8 cups parsley, chopped
- 2 cups cilantro, chopped
- 2 cups blueberries

Procedure:

1. Put all ingredients in the food processor and blend until smooth.
2. Pour the smoothies into the glasses.

Fresh Blackberries Smoothie

Servings: 4

Preparation Time: 10 minutes

Per Serving: 180 calories,3.3g protein, 12.1g carbohydrates, 14.9g fat, 6.1g fiber, 0mg cholesterol, 27mg sodium, 441mg potassium.

Ingredients:

- 2 cups parsley, chopped
- 2 cups blackberries
- 1 cup of coconut milk

Procedure:

1. First, blend all ingredients in the blender until smooth.
2. Serve the cooked smoothie with ice cubes.